ESSENTIAL GUIDE TO MELASMA

Comprehensive Strategies for Diagnosis, Treatment, and Management

DR. CASEY LOREN

DISCLAIMER

This book's content is only meant to be used for general informative purposes. Although the author has taken great care to ensure the content is accurate and thorough, no warranties or assurances on the information's accuracy, correctness, or reliability are provided. It is recommended that readers employ their own judgment and discretion when applying any material found in this book to their particular situation.

The information in this book is not intended to replace professional advice, nor is the author an expert in any of the subjects covered. It is recommended that readers consult with experienced professionals regarding any particular issues or concerns.

Any name that may be mentioned or referred in this book does not imply endorsement, recommendation, or relationship on the part of the author with any person, entity, good, website, or association. These references are made only for informational purposes and are not meant to be taken as recommendations or endorsements.

The information contained in this book may cause readers to suffer loss or damage, for which the author disclaims all obligation and accountability. The only people accountable for the decisions and actions taken by readers using the information presented are themselves.

Any names, characters, companies, locations, activities, occasions, and incidents referenced in this book are either made up or the result of the author's imagination. Any likeness to real people, living or dead, or to real things is entirely coincidental.

This book's content may change at any time, without prior notice, according to the author.

The onus is on the reader to verify whether there have been any updates or revisions.

The reader accepts the conditions of this disclaimer by reading this book. Please do not read this book or use its contents if you do not agree to these terms.

Table of Contents

CHAPTER 1

AN EXPLANATION AND SYNOPSIS OF MELASMA

A common skin disorder called melasma is characterized by the emergence of dark, uneven spots, especially on the face. These patches come in a variety of sizes and shapes and are frequently symmetrical. Usually appearing gradually, melasma may become more apparent after being exposed to the sun.

Melasma Causes and Triggers

Although the precise etiology of melasma is unknown, several factors, including hormone fluctuations, sun exposure, and genetic predisposition, are thought to play a role. Melasma can be brought on by hormonal changes, such as those that occur during pregnancy or when taking birth control pills. Sun exposure is particularly important because ultraviolet (UV) radiation stimulates melanocytes, which are the cells that give skin its color.

Melasma Types and Variants

Based on its distribution and appearance, melasma can be classified into several categories. Among these are dermal melasma, in which pigment is found deeper in the skin, and epidermal melasma, which is characterized by superficial pigment deposits. The features of both dermal and epidermal kinds are combined in mixed melasma.

Prevalence and Epidemiology

While it can afflict men as well, melasma is more frequently observed in women, especially those with darker skin tones. It is common in areas with strong sunshine and impacts people from different ethnic origins.

Risk Elements Linked to Melasma

Hormonal changes, sun exposure, family history, and certain drugs or cosmetics that may make the skin more sensitive to UV radiation are risk factors for developing melasma.

Effect on Life Quality

A person's quality of life may be greatly impacted by melasma, which can lead to emotional discomfort, problems with self-esteem, and difficulties interacting with others. Because the illness is noticeable on the face, people may feel self-conscious and decide to seek therapy as a result.

Differential diagnosis and diagnosis

Melasma diagnosis usually requires a complete skin examination as well as a medical history. To determine the skin's pigmentation level, use a Wood's light. To differentiate melasma from other pigmentation disorders such as post-inflammatory hyperpigmentation or lentigines, differential diagnosis is crucial.

Why Getting a Professional Diagnosis Is Important

For melasma, a professional diagnosis is essential because self-diagnosis might result in the wrong course of treatment and even make the problem worse. A dermatologist is qualified to identify melasma with accuracy and to suggest the best course of action.

Emotional and Psychological Impacts

Melasma can have significant psychological and emotional impacts on one's self-esteem, body image, and general well-being. Melasma sufferers may exhibit avoidance behaviors linked to their looks, anxiety, or depression.

Present Studies and Progress in the Understanding of Melasma

Understanding the underlying mechanisms of melasma, including the roles of hormones, genetics, and environmental variables, is the subject of ongoing research. The results of treatment for melasma sufferers are still becoming better thanks to developments in topical drugs, laser therapy, and chemical peels.

Healthcare providers may offer patients comprehensive care and support that addresses both the physical and emotional components of melasma by having a thorough awareness of the condition's intricacies.

CHAPTER 2

THE CAUSES AND PREVENTION OF MELASMA

Sun Exposure and UV Radiation:

These two factors are major contributors to the development of melasma. Melasma patches may appear or worsen as a result of ultraviolet light stimulating melanocytes, the skin's pigment-producing cells. Use high-SPF broad-spectrum sunscreen, find shade during the hottest parts of the day, and cover yourself with hats and sunglasses to avoid this.

Hormonal Factors (Pregnancy, Hormone Therapy):

Hormonal changes brought on by pregnancy and hormone therapy may aggravate melasma. Elevated estrogen levels during pregnancy can stimulate melanocytes, resulting in the appearance of melasma, commonly known as the "mask of pregnancy." Similarly, hormone therapy, which includes hormone replacement therapy and birth control pills, can affect the synthesis of melanin. For people who are susceptible to melasma, it is imperative to speak with a medical practitioner about controlling their hormone swings.

Genetic Predisposition and Family History:

Melasma is largely influenced by genetics. Melasma runs in families, so those who have a history of it are more likely to get it themselves. By being aware of this inherited tendency, people can take preventative and management actions to avoid and manage melasma. These actions include using sunscreen religiously, maintaining a healthy skincare regimen, and consulting a specialist to discuss treatment choices.

Ingredients and Skincare Products to Steer Clear of A few ingredients and skincare products can make melasma worse. Certain scents, strong exfoliants, and hydroquinone are examples of ingredients that might exacerbate uneven pigmentation by inflaming the skin. Choose skincare products that are mild and non-irritating for sensitive skin, and stay away from products that can exacerbate melasma.

Lifestyle Factors (Diet, Stress, Sleep):

Poor diet, stress, and sleep deprivation can affect hormone levels and hasten the onset of melasma. Stress management strategies like deep breathing, eating a well-balanced, nutrient- and antioxidant-rich diet, and getting enough sleep each night will improve general skin health and possibly lessen factors that lead to melasma.

Environmental Factors (Heat, Pollution):

Melasma can be made worse by environmental factors like heat and pollution. Heat can activate melanocytes, and pollution can cause oxidative stress. These triggers can be reduced by using antioxidants to shield the skin from environmental aggressors and by keeping a cool, well-ventilated atmosphere.

Sun protection measures are very important since they can help prevent and manage melasma. This entails avoiding lengthy sun exposure, especially during peak hours, seeking shade, using protective clothes, and applying broad-spectrum sunscreen every day. It is imperative to wear sunscreen consistently, especially on overcast days or in the winter.

Antioxidants' Function in Prevention:

By scavenging free radicals and lowering oxidative stress on the skin, antioxidants are essential in the fight against melasma. Antioxidants such as niacinamide, vitamin C, and vitamin E can be used in skincare regimens to assist promote general skin health and prevent harm to the environment.

Steer Clear of Common Triggers in Daily Life:

In addition to sun exposure, controlling melasma requires steering clear of common triggers such as hormone changes, harsh skincare products, and environmental pollution. Melasma flare-ups can be avoided by being aware of environmental variables, skincare components, and lifestyle choices.

Advice for Preventing Melasma Recurrence:

The key to preventing melasma recurrence is to stick to a consistent skincare regimen that is specific to your skin type, use sunscreen every day, stay away from triggers, control your stress levels, and consult a specialist for advice on the right therapies. Regular visits to a dermatologist can also aid in monitoring skin health and quickly addressing any issues.

CHAPTER 3

SUBTYPES AND CLINICAL PRESENTATION

Melasma, which can be classified as either epidermal, dermal, or mixed, is a common condition of acquired hyperpigmentation that is characterized by sporadic patches of brown to grayish-brown pigmentation on skin areas exposed to sunlight. Three subtypes can be distinguished: mixed, dermal, and epidermal melasma. Brown pigmentation mostly in the epidermal layer is the hallmark of epidermal melasma, which is visible when examined with a Wood's lamp. Deeper dermal pigmentation is involved in dermal melasma, which frequently manifests as bluish-gray areas. Mixed melasma exhibits a mixture of brown and bluish-gray pigmentation, including characteristics of both epidermal and dermal forms.

Distribution and Characteristic Patterns:

Melasma usually appears symmetrically across the face, especially on the chin, upper lip, forehead, and cheeks. Depending on the individual, the distribution may differ significantly, but it frequently follows a distinctive pattern called centrofacial, malar, or mandibular. Affected areas of the face by centrofacial melasma include the chin, upper lip, forehead, and nose. Whereas mandibular melasma affects the jawline, malar melasma manifests on the cheeks.

Variations in Melasma Lesion Colour:

Melasma lesions can vary in color from light brown to dark brown or bluish-gray. This color difference is a result of the skin layers' depth of pigmentation. Dermal melasma has a bluish-gray appearance, but epidermal melasma is typically light to medium brown. These colors are combined in mixed melasma, which frequently appears as a mixture of light brown and bluish-gray areas.

Distinguishing Melasma from Other Skin Disorders:

Post-inflammatory hyperpigmentation, lentigines, and melasma-like medication reactions are some of the disorders that might mimic melasma. A complete medical history in addition to a clinical examination can help distinguish melasma from several other illnesses. In difficult cases, skin biopsies, dermoscopies, and Wood's lamp examinations can be used to obtain a reliable diagnosis.

Clinical Examination and Assessment Instruments:

Wood's lamp examination, which aids in differentiating between epidermal and dermal pigmentation, is one of the instruments dermatologists use to evaluate melasma during clinical examinations. The evaluation of pigment distribution and patterns is aided by dermoscopy. When screening out other illnesses or in atypical circumstances, a skin biopsy may be necessary.

Correct Diagnosis Is Essential for Efficient Treatment:

Timely diagnosis is essential for efficient treatment of melasma. Misdiagnosis might result in ineffective treatment and pigmentation worsening. To customize treatment plans and attain the best results, a thorough assessment that takes into account clinical presentation, distribution, and diagnostic resources is required.

Understanding Melasma Patterns in Different Skin Types:

Fitzpatrick skin types III to VI are more likely to experience melasma than other skin types.

However, melasma can occur in individuals with any skin type. Accurate detection of post-inflammatory hyperpigmentation is more difficult in darker skin types. Dermatologists need to be skilled in identifying melasma patterns on various skin types to offer individualized therapy.

Interactions between Photodamage and Melasma:

Prolonged sun exposure increases pigment production and melanocyte activity, which exacerbates melasma. In addition to causing melasma, photodamage also makes treatment outcomes more challenging. Therefore, photoprotection is essential to managing melasma to avoid UV-induced pigmentation and enhance therapy response.

Effect of Hormonal Changes on Melasma Presentation:

Hormonal variables, especially in women, are important in the development of melasma.

Hormone replacement medication, pregnancy, oral contraceptives, and hormonal changes can all make melasma worse. The development and duration of melasma lesions are influenced by melanocyte activity and pigmentation, which is influenced by estrogen and progesterone.

The duration and recurrence of melasma lesions:

Melasma is frequently a chronic illness with flare-ups and remissions. Melasma lesions may continue to exist after therapy, necessitating ongoing care. Due to the chronic nature of melasma, factors like sun exposure, hormone fluctuations, and hereditary predisposition must be taken into consideration when providing continuous patient education and follow-up therapy.

To give patients with this difficult pigmentary illness complete care and better treatment outcomes, dermatologists must have a thorough understanding of all the facets of melasma, from its subtypes and distribution patterns to its interactions with hormonal shifts and photodamage.

CHAPTER 4

OPTIONS FOR MELASMA TREATMENT

Topical agents (azelaic acid, retinoid, and hydroquinone):

Topical treatments, which try to lighten hyperpigmented regions and control melanin synthesis, are frequently the initial line of treatment for melasma. As a gold standard for treating melasma, hydroquinone works by preventing the creation of melanin. However, because of possible adverse effects such as skin irritation and ochronosis with continuous use, it's important to utilize it carefully and under professional advice.

Adapalene and other retinoid-containing products function by increasing cell turnover and improving the absorption of other lightening agents. Although they work well, they could make your skin sensitive, especially in the beginning.

Another choice with anti-inflammatory and melanin-inhibiting qualities is azelaic acid. It works best when combined with other agents and is generally well-tolerated.

Chemical Peels (Trichloroacetic Acid, Glycolic Acid):

Applying a solution to the skin to exfoliate and enhance its appearance is known as a chemical peel. Gentle glycolic acid peels can help with melasma by decreasing pigmentation and increasing skin turnover. Stronger and potentially useful in more extreme situations, trichloroacetic acid (TCA) peels need to be applied carefully and require aftercare to avoid problems like hyperpigmentation or scarring.

Q-switched, fractional, and IPL laser therapy:

Different wavelengths are used in laser therapy to target melanin in the skin. Melanin can be efficiently targeted with Q-switched lasers, such as Q-switched Nd: YAG or alexandrite lasers, without causing harm to the surrounding tissue. Similar to fractional CO_2 or erbium lasers, fractional lasers induce controlled damage to promote pigment dispersion and skin remodeling. Another approach that targets hemoglobin and melanin and is versatile in treating a range of skin problems is Intense Pulsed Light (IPL).

Oral Medications (Tranexamic Acid, Oral Antioxidants):

When taken orally, tranexamic acid can help suppress the production of melanin and decrease melanocyte activity. For best effects, it is frequently used in conjunction with other therapies. Oral antioxidants that improve skin health and lower oxidative stress, such as glutathione, vitamin C, and vitamin E, can help control melasma.

Sequential treatment approaches and combination therapies:

Combining several techniques can improve results and treat various melasma features. For best results, for instance, a series of topical medications, chemical peels, and laser therapy may be applied one after the other. A methodical strategy is used in sequential treatments, introducing stronger therapies progressively as needed while keeping an eye on skin response and reducing adverse effects.

Sun Protection Is Crucial During Treatment:

Since UV rays can cause or exacerbate pigmentation, protecting oneself from the sun is essential for managing melasma. Patients should avoid peak sun hours, wear protective clothes and accessories, and apply broad-spectrum sunscreen with SPF 30 or greater every day. It is better to use sunscreens with physical blockers like titanium dioxide or zinc oxide because of their softer composition and a wider spectrum of protection.

Patient Instruction and Adherence:

Making educated decisions and encouraging treatment compliance are two benefits of educating patients about the origins, triggers, and available treatments for melasma. Patients should be aware of the significance of regular treatment compliance, using sunscreen, and scheduling follow-up sessions to track their progress and modify their treatment plan as necessary.

Considering Hormonal Effects in Treatment Regimens:

Melasma can be influenced by hormonal variables, such as hormone replacement treatment or pregnancy. It's critical to modify therapy regimens to account for hormonal swings or imbalances. The all-encompassing strategy may include things like avoiding hormonal triggers, modifying oral contraceptives, or adding hormone-regulating drugs.

Controlling Treatment Expectations:

To prevent disappointment and guarantee patient happiness throughout melasma therapy, it is essential to set reasonable expectations. Progress could be gradual, and total resolution isn't always possible. Reiterating steady improvement, regular treatment compliance, and continuous upkeep can help control expectations and improve therapy results.

Strategies for Long-Term Maintenance:

For melasma to sustain effects and stop reoccurring, long-term care is frequently necessary. The continuous application of topical medications, sporadic chemical peels or laser treatments, regular sun protection routines, and lifestyle adjustments to reduce triggers are examples of long-term maintenance techniques. Scheduling routine follow-up visits with medical professionals enables ongoing monitoring and necessary modifications to the maintenance plan.

CHAPTER 5

LIFESTYLE ADJUSTMENTS FOR THE MANAGEMENT OF MELASMA

Nutrition and Dietary Advice for Skin Health

In addition to improving general health, a well-balanced diet high in vitamins, minerals, and antioxidants can help with skin disorders like melasma. Throughout your meals, include an abundance of fruits, vegetables, whole grains, lean proteins, and healthy fats. Antioxidant-rich foods like almonds, leafy greens, and berries can help prevent oxidative stress and improve the health of your skin.

Techniques for Stress Management

Acquiring proficiency in stress management strategies is essential, as prolonged stress can either precipitate or worsen melasma. Try some relaxation exercises like yoga, tai chi, meditation, or deep breathing. Take part in enjoyable activities, get outside, and practice mindfulness to lower stress and enhance general well-being.

The Value of Consistent Sleep Habits

Getting enough sleep is crucial for managing melasma and maintaining healthy skin. Try to get between seven and nine hours of sleep every night. To encourage peaceful sleep and help skin regeneration, establish a soothing bedtime routine, create a comfortable sleep environment, and avoid screens and stimulating activities before bedtime.

The Effects of Exercise on Melasma

Frequent exercise improves general health, increases circulation, and lowers stress—all of which have an indirect positive impact on the management of melasma. Choose mild exercise regimens like swimming, cycling, or walking. When engaging in outdoor activities, try to limit your exposure to the sun. To protect your skin, wear sunscreen and protective gear.

Skincare Protocols for Skin Prone to Melasma

To effectively manage melasma, a mild skincare regimen is necessary. Use moisturizers appropriate for your skin type, non-abrasive exfoliants, and moderate cleansers. Include skin-brightening elements in your skincare regimen, such as licorice extract, vitamin C, niacinamide, and kojic acid. See a dermatologist for advice on specific skincare regimens.

Selecting Sunscreen and Makeup Products Sensibly

Select makeup products that are hypoallergenic and non-comedogenic, specially designed for

skin that is sensitive or prone to melasma. To protect against UVA and UVB radiation, use sunscreens with broad-spectrum protection (SPF 30 or higher) and physical blockers like titanium dioxide or zinc oxide. Every two hours, as well as after swimming or perspiring, reapply sunscreen.

Preventing Overexposure to Humidity and Heat

Consider taking measures to prevent overexposure to heat and humidity since these factors might aggravate melasma. When the sun is at its strongest, stay inside, use air conditioning or cooling fans, and when you are outside, wear light, breathable clothing and wide-brimmed hats. Keep your skin hydrated and cool to reduce flare-ups of melasma.

Advice for Effectively Handling Hormonal Changes

Melasma can be brought on by hormonal changes, such as those that occur during pregnancy or after taking hormone medication. For individualized hormone control plans, speak with medical professionals. Follow skincare guidelines, control stress, and lead a healthy lifestyle to help reduce hormonally associated melasma symptoms.

Including Holistic Methods in Everyday Life

Acupuncture, herbal medicines, and dietary supplements are examples of holistic approaches that can be used in addition to traditional therapy for melasma. For individualized advice, speak with licensed professionals with knowledge in holistic medicine. Use caution when using herbal supplements, and let your doctor know about any supplementary treatments you're doing.

Establishing a Helpful Environment for the Management of Melasma

Be in the company of a network of family, friends, and medical professionals who are sympathetic to your melasma adventure. Inform close ones about the illness, ask for emotional support when required, and work with medical specialists to create a thorough management plan that takes into account your particular requirements and objectives.

CHAPTER 6

EFFECTS ON THE MIND AND COPING MECHANISMS

Melasma's Emotional Impact on Self-Esteem

Melasma can have a major negative influence on self-esteem due to its obvious effects on the skin. People may experience self-consciousness, which can impair confidence and result in a bad body image. Reducing the emotional load can be accomplished by realizing that melasma is a common disorder influenced by a variety of circumstances, such as sun exposure and hormone fluctuations. Addressing the physical features of melasma, getting professional skincare advice, and investigating treatment options can also help improve self-esteem.

Managing Depression and Anxiety

Melasma can be accompanied by anxiety and despair because of how stressful it is to manage and how it affects looks. Practicing mindfulness, getting regular exercise, and leading a balanced lifestyle are examples of coping mechanisms. Getting therapy or counseling from mental health specialists can also give you important tools for efficiently managing depression and anxiety.

Asking Friends and Family for Support

Being honest about melasma with friends and family might help to build understanding and support. The emotional burden might be lighter and a supportive environment can be created by sharing feelings and experiences. Fostering empathy and significant support can also be achieved by educating close ones about melasma.

Self-talk That Is Positively Important

A key component of melasma coping is positive self-talk. Changing one's negative thoughts to positive ones can boost one's well-being and sense of self. Self-compassion exercises and an emphasis on one's abilities can help one adopt a more optimistic perspective.

Options for Counselling and Therapy

Getting professional treatment or counseling might help manage the emotional effects of melasma. Acceptance and commitment therapy (ACT) and cognitive-behavioral therapy (CBT) are useful strategies for overcoming negative thoughts and fostering resilience. These treatments provide specialized coping mechanisms for managing anxiety, depression, and stress.

Practices of Mindfulness and Meditation

Meditation and mindfulness techniques help people unwind, lower their stress levels, and become more self-aware. Including mindfulness in everyday activities can aid in the management of melasma-related emotions. Methods like mindfulness exercises, deep breathing, and meditation can promote mental health and induce a state of tranquility.

Taking Part in Online Communities or Support Groups

It can be empowering to connect with people going through similar struggles in online communities or support groups. In these communities, exchanging advice, encouragement, and experiences promotes a feeling of community and lessens feelings of loneliness. It also offers the chance to pick up coping mechanisms from peers.

Having Reasonable Expectations and Goals

It's crucial to have reasonable expectations and goals for your melasma therapy and self-care. It helps to know that melasma may need to be managed continuously to avoid disappointment and anger. Honoring modest victories and advancements helps keep one's spirits up and increases motivation.

Honouring Developments and Minor Wins

Acknowledging any advancement, regardless of its magnitude, is crucial in managing melasma. Recognizing accomplishments in skincare practices or emotional fortitude boosts confidence and positive behavior. Honoring significant accomplishments in the process of controlling melasma can be uplifting and empowering.

Accepting and loving oneself

Developing self-love and accepting self-care techniques are essential to managing melasma. Making skincare routines, healthy behaviors, and enjoyable and relaxing activities a priority all contribute to overall well-being. Acceptance, self-compassion, and treating oneself with kindness and respect are all necessary components in nurturing self-love.

In conclusion, treating the emotional effects of melasma necessitates a multifaceted strategy that includes self-care routines, constructive coping mechanisms, support networks, and expert advice. By adopting these techniques, people can manage the difficulties associated with melasma and promote their mental and emotional health.

CHAPTER 7

MELASMA IN CERTAIN GROUPS OF PEOPLE

Chloasma, or melasma in pregnancy:

Chloasma, sometimes referred to as the "mask of pregnancy," or melasma during pregnancy, is a common skin disorder marked by the development of hyperpigmented patches on the face. Usually, it's caused by hormonal fluctuations, especially elevated progesterone and estrogen levels, which can speed up the skin's synthesis of melanin.

Because there are fewer treatment options available, managing melasma in pregnant women requires caution to protect the developing fetus as well as the mother. Because of the possible hazards, topical medications containing hydroquinone, tretinoin, and some acids may not be recommended during pregnancy. As a safer alternative, moisturizing, mild cleaning, and sunscreen protection are frequently advised.

Pregnant women with melasma should see a dermatologist or other healthcare professional to ensure they receive the right advice and support during their pregnancy.

Paediatric Melasma and Its Treatments:

Although it is somewhat uncommon, melasma can occur in pediatric patients despite being more common in adults. Because pediatric skin is so fragile, treating pediatric melasma needs to be done with caution and gentleness.

Children's melasma can have a variety of underlying reasons, such as hormone imbalances, sun exposure, hereditary predisposition, or specific drugs. Compared to adult melasma, treatment options for pediatric melasma are usually more restricted and center on sun protection, mild skincare, and avoiding potential triggers.

Pediatric dermatologists frequently customize treatment regimens for their patients taking into account the child's age, underlying medical conditions, and the severity of the ailment. To assess progress and modify the treatment plan as necessary, routine follow-ups and monitoring are crucial.

Men's Melasma and Considerations Based on Gender:

Melasma affects both men and women, however it affects women more frequently. Gender differences may exist in the presentation and underlying reasons, though. Sun exposure, genetic predisposition, hormone imbalances, and specific drugs are frequently linked to melasma in men.

Men's melasma management follows the same guidelines as women's, which include avoiding recognized triggers, wearing sunscreen, and using moderate skincare products. However, given that men and women have different skin physiologies and hormonal profiles, treatment strategies might need to be modified.

Men with melasma can benefit from individualized treatment programs that address their unique requirements and concerns, taking gender-specific factors into account, by consulting with a dermatologist.

Melasma in Various Skin Types and Ethnic Groups:

Although melasma can affect people of all races and skin types, Fitzpatrick skin types III-VI, which include people with more pigment in their skin, are more likely to experience it.

Ethnic groups may exhibit varied patterns of melasma, with some exhibiting more prominent pigmentation or involvement of distinct facial areas. It is essential to comprehend these differences to properly customize treatment regimens.

Different ethnicities and skin types may require different topical treatments for melasma, such as hydroquinone, retinoids, and antioxidants, in addition to rigorous sun protection measures. When creating treatment plans for various populations, dermatologists take into account variables such as skin sensitivity, reaction to therapies, and possible side effects.

Postmenopausal Women's Melasma:

Hormone changes that postmenopausal women may encounter may have an impact on the onset or aggravation of melasma. Particularly during this time of life, changes in estrogen levels may contribute to the development or aggravation of melasma.

Postmenopausal women with melasma need to manage the condition with a multifaceted approach that takes hormones, UV exposure, skincare practices, and possible treatments into account. To reduce the effect on melasma, hormone replacement treatment (HRT) may need to be assessed and modified in cooperation with medical professionals.

Depending on the needs and objectives of each patient, topical treatments, chemical peels, laser therapy, and other interventions may be taken into consideration. Monitoring progress and maximizing treatment results require routine skin examinations and follow-ups.

Patients with Hormonal Imbalances and Melasma:

Melasma can develop or worsen as a result of hormonal abnormalities, such as those caused by thyroid diseases or polycystic ovarian syndrome (PCOS). Hormone levels, such as those of estrogen, progesterone, and androgens, can be affected by these imbalances, and this can have an impact on the skin's ability to produce melanin.

In addition to standard melasma treatments, managing melasma in people with hormone imbalances frequently includes treating the underlying hormonal problems. To successfully regulate hormonal variables and optimize therapy outcomes, dermatologists and endocrinologists may need to collaborate.

Based on individual assessments and medical history, combination therapy that targets both hormone regulation and skin pigmentation, such as topical medicines, oral medications, and lifestyle modifications, may be suggested.

Patients with medical comorbidities and melasma:

Individuals who have specific medical conditions together, such as diabetes, liver illness, or autoimmune disorders, may be more likely to develop or experience consequences from melasma. These disorders may affect several physiological functions, such as the regulation of pigmentation and the health of the skin.

Dermatologists, primary care physicians, and specialists in charge of the underlying medical disorders must collaborate to manage melasma in patients with medical comorbidities. It can be required to do thorough evaluations that include blood work, prescription reviews, and medical histories to customize treatment regimens and handle any possible interactions or contraindications.

To minimize side effects, assure treatment efficacy, and address any changes in the patient's overall health status, close observation, and routine follow-ups are necessary.

Transgender People's Melasma:

Transgender people may be affected by melasma, and treatment options may differ depending on skin type, hormone medication, and personal health concerns. The production of melanin and skin pigmentation can be affected by hormone therapy, especially treatments using estrogen or testosterone, which may affect the development or severity of melasma.

When creating individualized treatment programs for transgender patients with melasma, dermatologists consider treatment preferences, skin sensitivity, and hormone medication regimens. Commonly advised tactics include using sunscreen, practicing gentle skincare, and applying topical medications as needed. Hormone therapy modifications are also frequently suggested.

To guarantee thorough care and the best possible treatment results, open communication and cooperation between dermatologists and transgender healthcare professionals are crucial.

Melasma in Senior Citizens:

Even while it may manifest differently in older patients than in younger ones, melasma can nonetheless develop or persist in them. Melasma in older patients can be influenced by various factors, including age, medication use, cumulative sun exposure, and hormonal changes.

Personalized strategies that take into account things like skin fragility, comorbid medical disorders, and possible drug interactions are necessary for managing melasma in older people. Sun protection, coupled with moderate skincare techniques and judicious topical treatment use, continue to be cornerstones of management.

Based on the unique features of each patient's skin and the intended course of treatment, dermatologists may suggest procedures such as fractional laser therapy, chemical peels, or microneedling. To maximize results and preserve senior patients' skin health, regular evaluations, and plan modifications are crucial.

Customising Care for Particular Groups:

Treatment for melasma must take into account the particular requirements, traits, and difficulties faced by particular groups. This covers elements including age, gender, skin type, ethnicity, hormonal balance, past medical history, and preferred course of therapy.

Dermatologists use a wide range of treatment modalities, such as oral medications (like tranexamic acid), chemical peels, laser therapies (like fractional lasers, Q-switched lasers), topical agents (like hydroquinone, retinoids, and azelaic acid), and customized combination approaches.

Based on the patient's response to the medication, any adverse effects, and modifications to their lifestyle or health, the treatment plan may alter over time. Effective management of melasma in certain groups requires regular follow-ups, patient education, and coordination with other healthcare practitioners.

CHAPTER 8

DEVELOPMENTS IN THE STUDY OF MELASMA

New Treatment Strategies Under Investigation:

Scientists are investigating cutting-edge strategies for treating melasma that go beyond conventional medicine. This involves looking for novel substances, combinations, and technological advancements that can provide safer and more efficient melasma management options. These strategies might focus on melanogenesis inhibition, anti-inflammatory effects, or melanocyte modulation to target particular facets of melasma pathophysiology.

Precision medicine and targeted therapies:

These fields have been made possible by our growing understanding of the molecular mechanisms underlying melasma. These methods seek to customize treatment plans according to patient-specific traits such as skin type, genetics, and the underlying mechanisms causing melasma. To provide more specialized and targeted treatment approaches, researchers are focusing on certain targets, such as inflammatory cascades or pathways involved in melanin formation.

The identification of biomarkers and prognostic

parameters is of utmost importance in the prediction of melasma therapy response, disease progression, and personalized care. Numerous molecular markers, genetic signatures, hormonal profiles, and environmental factors that may affect the onset and course of melasma are being studied by researchers. Gaining knowledge about these indicators and variables may improve prognosis evaluations and enable more focused therapies.

Genetic Research on Melasma Susceptibility Genes:

Research on melasma susceptibility genes has provided information about the genetic propensity that underlies this disorder. Through deciphering the genetic components that lead to melasma, scientists are revealing the complex interactions of heredity, environment, and hormones. This information advances our understanding of the pathophysiology of melasma and creates opportunities for targeted genetic-based therapies.

Developments in Topical Delivery Systems:

By enhancing the effectiveness, safety, and patient compliance with topical medications, advancements in topical delivery systems are transforming the management of melasma. These developments include liposomal delivery, nanoencapsulation, microneedle technology, and other novel formulations intended to improve drug administration, target certain skin layers, and increase skin penetration for improved therapeutic results.

The potential of stem cell-based therapeutics in regulating melanocyte activity, skin regeneration, and pigmentation modification is being investigated in the rapidly developing field of stem cell-related melasma care. Promising paths for the development of innovative therapies that address the underlying causes of melasma and support long-term skin renewal and pigment regulation are provided by stem cell research.

Immunological Understanding of the Complex Pathogenesis of Melasma:

Developments in immunological research have shed light on the roles that immune dysregulation, inflammatory mediators, and immune cell interactions play in the formation and persistence of melasma. To treat the inflammatory part of melasma and create targeted immunomodulatory medicines, it is imperative to comprehend the immunological features of the illness.

Integrative medicine and alternative therapies are becoming more and more popular in the management of melasma since they provide alternate methods to traditional medical treatments. This includes acupuncture, dietary changes, botanical extracts, stress-reduction methods, and other holistic therapies that try to treat the various factors—such as oxidative stress, hormone imbalances, and psychological influences—that contribute to melasma.

Patient-reported Outcomes:

These outcomes are essential to the study of melasma because they shed light on how the condition affects patients' quality of life, emotional stability, and satisfaction with their treatments. Including patient viewpoints, preferences, and experiences facilitates the creation of patient-centered care plans, enhances treatment compliance, and provides a comprehensive evaluation of the efficacy of interventions.

Prospects for Future Directions and Potential Breakthroughs:

Research on melasma appears to have promising futures in terms of personalized medicines, diagnostic tools, and treatment methods. The field of melasma management is about to undergo a revolution thanks to emerging technologies including tailored medication delivery systems, genetics, regenerative medicine, and artificial intelligence in dermatology.

Working together, researchers, physicians, industry partners, and patient advocacy organizations can make significant progress toward ground-breaking discoveries and enhance the quality of life for melasma patients.

CHAPTER 9

CLINICAL SCENARIOS AND CASE STUDIES

Pregnancy-Related Melasma Management

Hormonal variations cause melasma during pregnancy, commonly referred to as the "mask of pregnancy," to present special complications. Pregnancy-safe topical medicines like azelaic acid and vitamin C, physical barriers like hats, and high-SPF sunscreen are all part of management. Avoiding procedures like laser therapy is also part of the plan. Counseling and regular monitoring are essential.

Patients with Dark Skin Receiving Treatment for Melasma

To prevent post-inflammatory hyperpigmentation, care must be taken when treating melasma in people with darker skin tones.

Topical medications (such as hydroquinone, kojic acid, and retinoids), mild chemical peels (like glycolic acid), and laser procedures (such as Nd: YAG lasers) are among the options. It's imperative to take a customized approach and closely monitor any negative consequences.

Success Stories of Combination Therapy

When it comes to managing melasma, combination therapies—such as applying topical medications in addition to laser or chemical peels—often produce superior outcomes. Success stories highlight calculated blends that meet specific requirements while striking a balance between effectiveness, safety, and tolerability.

Handling Cases with Resistant Melasma

A complete strategy is necessary for situations of resistant melasma, which may involve sophisticated therapies such as fractional laser resurfacing, microneedling, or combination laser therapies. Effective management of resistant patients necessitates controlling patient expectations, ensuring adherence to treatment programs, and doing frequent follow-ups.

Coping Mechanisms and Psychological Effects

Beyond just its physical manifestations, melasma also has an impact on one's quality of life and self-esteem. Cognitive-behavioral treatment, support groups, cosmetic concealment techniques, and patient education are all examples of coping mechanisms. Holistic care requires not only clinical management but also psychological well-being treatment.

Extended Upkeep and Monitoring

Long-term care includes regular chemical peels, maintenance laser treatments, ongoing topical medication application (such as hydroquinone or retinoids), and sun protection measures. Frequent check-ins track development, swiftly address relapses and modify treatment plans as necessary to achieve long-term results.

Clinical Scenario: Melasma and Hormonal Influences

Melasma is greatly influenced by hormonal factors, such as pregnancy or the use of oral contraceptives. Effective management of melasma requires knowledge of hormonal pathways, modification of treatment during changes in hormones, and consideration of alternate therapies, such as topical non-hormonal medicines.

Clinical Situation: Including Lifestyle Adjustments

Complementing therapeutic care of melasma is integrating lifestyle improvements such as stress reduction strategies, nutritious nutrition, getting enough sleep, and avoiding triggers (hot and sun). Lifestyle modifications promote general well-being and improve therapeutic results.

Clinical Scenario: Recurrence and Relapse of Melasma

Recurrence and relapse of melasma are frequent problems. Long-term maintenance treatments, consistent use of sun protection, frequent check-ups, and quick action at the first indications of recurrence are some strategies. For recurrent situations, combination therapies and customized strategies could be required.

Clinical Setting: Patient Instruction and Adherence

Teaching patients about the causes, symptoms, and available treatments for melasma is essential. Optimizing outcomes can be achieved by regular counseling sessions, visual aids, and clear communication that enhance understanding and promote commitment to treatment regimens.

CHAPTER 10

RESOURCES AND ASSISTANCE FOR PATIENTS

Locating Dermatologists and Specialists Who Are Qualified

Selecting the best dermatologist or melasma specialist requires taking into account several factors. Seek out experts who have dealt with pigmentation issues such as melasma. Dermatologists who are board-certified frequently possess specialized training in these fields. To locate licensed doctors in your area, look through listings from associations such as the American Academy of Dermatology.

Resources and Websites for Patient Education

Effective patient education is essential for melasma management. Trusted sources such as the Melasma Society or the American Academy of Dermatology (AAD) can offer thorough information about the condition, available treatments, and skincare regimen advice. Melasma research updates and scientific articles can be found on websites such as UpToDate and PubMed.

Associations for Assistance and Advocacy

Advocacy and support groups can help establish connections with those going through comparable struggles. For those with melasma, the National Organisation for Rare Disorders (NORD) and the American Melasma Association may provide forums, information, and support.

Social media groups and online forums

Social media groups and online forums can offer a space for exchanging advice and experiences. Social media platforms such as Reddit, Facebook groups, or specialty forums on sites like PatientsLikeMe or Inspire can be helpful. But always double-check information from these sources with your physician.

Melasma Awareness Events and Campaigns

Public awareness about melasma is increased through campaigns and events. During May, which is Skin Cancer Awareness Month, organizations such as the American Academy of Dermatological or nearby dermatological clinics may organize campaigns, webinars, or events.

Programs for Financial Assistance in Treatment

Programs for financial support can be available to assist with the expense of treating melasma. Certain pharmaceutical companies provide discounts or patient assistance programs for prescription drugs. For those in need of financial assistance, healthcare providers and nonprofit organizations might also offer grants or other resources.

Instruments to Monitor Melasma Development

Monitoring melasma progression is crucial to assessing how well a treatment is working. Apps such as SkinVision or MySkinPal can be used to track skincare regimens and keep an eye on pigmentation changes. Documenting progress or flare-ups can also be accomplished by keeping a picture diary or journal.

Self-help techniques and coping mechanisms

People with melasma may find that their quality of life is enhanced by coping mechanisms and self-help techniques. Sun protection measures (such as hats and sunscreen), mild skincare regimens, stress-reduction methods (such as yoga and meditation), and asking for help from family members or mental health specialists can all be helpful.

Testimonials from Patients and Success Stories

Testimonials from patients and success stories can inspire and give hope. Patient support groups and websites such as RealSelf frequently share success stories from people with melasma. However since each person's experience is different, seek the counsel of medical experts for individualized guidance.

Patient Empowerment for Improved Melasma Handling

Education, assistance, and resource availability are all necessary for patient empowerment. Encourage patients to learn as much as they can about their illness, to ask questions when they have appointments, and to work with medical professionals to develop treatment strategies.

Advocating for oneself and getting second opinions as necessary to guarantee thorough care are other aspects of empowerment.